MUSING ALONG THE WAY

Tears, Lies, and Fresh Fruit Pies

VOLUME 1: 1997–2001

MARTHA JOHNSON

PEARL MEADOW PRESS

ISBN: 9780984304820
Copyright 2011 by Martha Johnson
First Printing: May 2011

This book was printed in the United States of America by Lightning Source.
Published by Pearl Meadow Press, 255 Pearl Street, South Hadley, MA 01075
To order additional copies, call 413-532-2579, or email: mjggdi@comcast.net

Cover Photo by Harry Lavo
Graphic Design and Layout: Persona

Note: The preface and poems from the years 1997– 2001 were previously
published in June 2002 as *Musing Along the Way: A Woman's Journey Looking at
Her Life Through the Lens of Chronic Illness* by Martha Johnson Gilburg

Library of Congress Control Number: 2011900444

WHAT PEOPLE SAY

Martha Johnson's poems offer us a straightforward look at life's difficulties, struggles, blessings and joys. She doesn't flinch from taking a forward-looking view at what, for some, would be touchy subjects. We're the richer because of it.

–SEAN VERNON, Musician, Songwriter, Poet, Teacher

Martha Johnson has written a book about accepting illness and loss. In poems that are intensely personal and yet very familiar to anyone undergoing the same trials, she has recorded the bumpy road from fighting the inevitable effects of illness to living her life in such a way as to no longer feel limited. This book is a "must read" for anyone looking to understand those who live with chronic disease.

–MAGGIE HARLING, MD, Principal author, "So, you have MS. What's next?"

To those who value and appreciate the concept of the well-examined life, Martha Johnson offers a gift of wisdom and guidance. Her "musings" give expression to what many women feel at midlife even if they are not facing a life-altering medical diagnosis. In fearlessly sharing her personal trials and challenges, she leads the reader down a path to discovering one's own resurrection of hope and lightness of being.

–DANA MULLER, DMA, JD

As the author tries to come to terms with herself, her circumstances and her experiences, she acknowledges the voice of the poet within—a voice that surprises her, but a voice she wishes to learn to trust. We can only thank her for sharing these musings with us, as guides to reflection for our own journeys.

–MARGARITA SOROCK, PhD

DEDICATED TO

Compassionate doctors

Healers too many to name

Rudy and Sharon and the Gestalt Class of 2001

Dominique Desrochers, DC, who gave me hope

All those ready to claim their inner healer

CONTENTS

FOREWORD

Martha Johnson Gilburg did not plan this journey. She has little say in the itinerary. Her 'musings' portray a personal voyage to explore, re-define and become comfortable with her new self with chronic illness. Multiple sclerosis (MS) had to be recognized as one, among many, of her life's ventures.

In the last several decades, gains have been made in our understanding of the clinical presentation and pathophysiology of multiple sclerosis. There are more treatment options now. However, what triggers this auto-immune cascade remains unclear. There is no definitive diagnostic test. No two patients have exactly the same course. There is no known cure. So we, as neurologists, can gather data to diagnose, initiate maintenance therapy and offer support services along the way.

But we cannot answer with certainty many questions. "Why do I have this?" "What will MS mean for me on a day to day basis?" "What can I expect five or ten years from now?"

Therefore the majority of people diagnosed with MS must walk along a path of uncertainty and define this new territory for themselves — only then can the rest of living continue.

In "Musing Along the Way," Martha Johnson Gilburg has done just this with a voice that resonates for all who live with chronic illness.

Dawn M. Pearson, MD
October, 2001

PREFACE

My diagnosis of Multiple Sclerosis was pronounced in October 1997. I had been having symptoms of "something very strange" since 1996. Co-ownership with my husband of our small consulting business — was becoming an increasingly stressful proposition. In 1998, we engaged in intensive couples therapy. In June of 2000, we packed up two condos and our small business and moved from Maryland to Massachusetts a very stressful six months on either side of that date. That summer, my limp became visible to all. When my symptoms were still invisible to others, I had learned to announce, in the groups I led or attended, that I had been diagnosed with MS. Most often, it was reassuring to hear from people who would seek me out and share their own experience and resources. Encouraged, I dealt with my initial hesitancy to reveal myself and looked forward to the treasures that would come in response to my simple statement, "I have been diagnosed with MS."

Nine months after the move, I was feeling more relaxed and settled. I had found wonderful doctors and healers in western New England. My relationship with my husband was moving into the dark days that I knew could precede the dawn. Not so pleasant — but actually necessary.

One day, at the beginning of March 2001, these musings started to flow unbidden. Without thought about publication, I sat down at the computer and recorded what came. Again, after nine months, they have been compiled and basically organized themselves. They appear as my testimony to the trials, insights and adventures dealing with a chronic illness with no known cause and no known cure. The attendant stresses that both exacerbate this dis-ease and flow from it also receive their due in these pages.

(continued)

I seemed to have been documenting my passage through to a new life, with a chronic condition as one of my companions. It is something I now want to share:

- The confusion of the early days while seeking a path
- Anger at a system which purports to be about health
- Naming and addressing the pain of stress at home
- The continuing difficulty of changing my ways
- Coping with loss and limitation, and
- Finding my own peace and perspective.

It truly has been an adventure for me — often sad, often confusing, amazingly joyous, too. These musings document the moments of pain, joy, anger and insight, and put this 5-year journey in perspective — for now.

The "for now" is the reason I labeled this "Book One". Over the last 20 years, pages of notes for other books previously started and aborted have multiplied themselves in my basement storage. I am aware that, in those days, attempting to say something meaningful, I always came to a place where I doubted that my own voice belonged in public space. I projected my awareness of how much I didn't know onto others. I feared I would be judged for what I didn't know, rather than appreciated for my hard won insights.

I am a different woman now. And this has been a reasonably effortless process. While still aware of my own hesitancy to speak coherently about a journey that is not yet complete, I no longer intimidate myself with the fact that I don't yet know what I will know in the years to come. I accept that in the next five years I will have some new perspectives about these years and may want to refine my current understandings with additional reflections.

The label of "Book One" is my gift to myself. I am giving myself permission to be imperfect and incomplete, and still offer my voice to the world.

After all, this is now, and I am here. This is what I think and feel today. For me, these musings, as they have emerged, have helped make meaning of this life that is mine. Perhaps my expression in these pages will encourage those of you with other life challenges, to give voice to your own story, as imperfect, incomplete, and chaotic as it may seem to be.

To have gained the ability to feel more deeply, think more clearly, and be more joyful, have not been small gifts of this process. My journey is not over, and I am not cured. However, I believe I am healing. There is a difference. Since I hold that "healing" must precede "curing", I choose to keep adventuring. This is as good as it gets — for now.

Enjoy...

Martha Johnson Gilburg
December, 2001

THE GRAND ADVENTURE

HEY, I'VE GOT A CHOICE!

When there is no known cause

And no known cure,

The healing journey gets to be a

GRAND ADVENTURE!

MS

Through my first marriage I became
Martha Spice.
For 30 years I initialed myself "MS".

And then, I got MS.
A friend pointed out that I should
Perhaps no longer sign myself "MS".

I took the advice.
Why add unnecessary affirmation to who I am
With a label I don't want?

Martha Johnson Gilburg

ON BEING AUTO IMMUNE

More than occasionally I ponder
How come the part of me that is supposed to protect me,
Has suddenly turned to attack.
Biology and physiology can track the phenomenon
But not the source.

Maybe the answer can be glimpsed
Exploring the metaphor.
What part of me is attacking what other part of me?
And how does that serve me?

Bringing More Joy...

My doctor said: "This condition is
Made worse by stress."

As I imagine most conditions are.

She was a role model in that
She had healed herself
From the very same condition.

"First," she said, "we start by eliminating
The stressors on the body,
And providing proper nourishment.
Eat healthy, get rest, drink water, exercise,
Take your vitamins."

No more lip service or excuses —
It's got to be a regimen!

"Next," she added, "we evaluate your work.
Do less of what you feel you have to do
Do more of what you love,
Spend fewer hours 'working'."

"Finally, eliminate the activities and relationships
Which don't nourish you,
And bring more joy into the life you live."

Sooo, I invite you to my bathroom gallery
For newly created joyous watercolors.

Now, months later,
I learn that she had
Taken her own advice
And divorced her husband.
She seems quite happy.

Another Way to Think About Chronic Illness...

It's a signal that something needs to be said.
The silencing of myself can go on no longer.

Yes, writing my truth has been
A self-administered emergency room treatment.
A desperate and final strategy for one silenced woman.

Retrospective

An eight year old Brownie Scout,
Got sick at overnight camp and had to go home.
Her fever down, she tearfully begged to stay home.
Her well intentioned mother, believing
That this now 'well' child belonged at camp,
Overruled her pleadings and sent her back.

The little girl made a logical decision for that time.
"Never again will I admit my hurt.
Never again will I risk revealing what I really need."
And, in an eight year old's way,
She asked herself a question,
"If I must silence my deepest self,
Who must I be in the world?"

WHERE IS MY ANGER?

I wondered where the anger was…
Five years of busyness
Running a business,
Attending to health,
A household move,
Dealing with a less than compassionate health care system,
Trying to be rational about an MS condition that came to visit
And stayed beyond welcome.

Yes, I've been angry at myself, my husband, my clients,
The Western medical model,
But never at the illness…
Curious…
Until today…
I felt serious anger at my MS
Wordlessly pass through my whole body…
And vanish!

"Next time, please stay and let's have a chat.
You <u>certainly</u> deserve to be heard."

HEALTH CARE HAVOC

Caution: Sharp Curves Ahead

Some of these musings are angry and whining, perhaps even raw and rude. This is the way I felt for a long time, and to some extent, still do. I am intensely angry at a system of health care constructed to fit a Western medical paradigm in which doctors, trained in narrow specialties, expect to know what's best for me, better than I.

What is less expressed here is my deep gratitude to the many compassionate doctors and healers who held my hand along the way. They helped me navigate the uncertainties, and risked themselves daily to believe in, and create, a new paradigm for health care.

Ultimately, I hope to find an equal amount of strength and courage to constructively stand for a system we all deserve.

A True Story

It wasn't a "right to health" state
Where doctors have wider latitude
In which to exercise
Their professional judgment.

An MD, an ND, and a dentist,
All appropriately credentialed by US institutions,
All compassionate healers with broader views,
Are today being harassed and fined
By their own State Boards.

I am sad for me,
I am sad for them,
I am angry at our system.

I wish intelligent, consenting adults
Might have the right to choose.

A National Shame

It's depleting, discouraging, and
Should be an indictable offense
That I must use the energy
I need for my healing
To battle my health care system
For the care I think I require.

OVER AT THE HMO

He was a very nice primary care doctor, who
Did listen to my plans for my own treatment, and
Tried to be supportive.
He referred me to a second neurologist for a second opinion.

He was a very nice neurologist
And explained the three AMA certified treatments for my
    condition.
"Of course there is no cure, but one of these may be helpful."
In response to my question about diet, he said:
"There is no research to indicate that diet makes
    any difference at all."

On another occasion,
My extremely nice primary care doctor
Asked me, " What is acupuncture anyway?"
He was kind enough to refer me, at my request,
To the newly appointed Coordinator of Alternative Approaches.

She was a very nice doctor of alternative approaches
Who introduced herself as being in charge of the "weird ward"
She suggested meditation.
She did approve my request for treatment with acupuncture
But only with the less experienced practitioners who
Have the patience to ally themselves with the HMO bureaucracy.

She was a very nice and responsive acupuncturist
She had to send complicated reports about how well I responded.
They paid her 3 months late and she never complained.
She documented the forward progress that was necessary to receive
Continued authorization for treatment.
She was as creative as she could be,
Considering my condition is chronic, and requires a maintenance plan rather than a fix.

LOOKING FOR THE EXPERT

I went to a respected local pharmacist
Who held a theory that many of my symptoms
Might be explained by an overgrowth of yeast.
He recommended the very rigorous Candida Diet
No sugar, no wheat, no fat,
No anything as far as I could tell.

I embraced that rigorous diet–for a while — and felt better.

After a few months I discovered that a well known doctor
Truly believed that MS could be halted.
Part of his regimen was a diet WITH fat and plenty of red meat.

I embraced that diet — for a while — and felt more energetic.

There were several other iterations of diets
Which made good sense in themselves,
But were quite contradictory to each other.

It was hard to shift my own believing about what is right
With an exact opposite prescription.
Hard to see how the experts who are in charge of advising
Could be in such disagreement.
I'd call that a time of Diet Dizziness and Unwelcome Whiplash.
I ultimately cleared my confusion.
I made myself the expert and trusted my own experience.
There was no other way.

I feel better. Period.

BRING BACK COMMON SENSE

In addition to the stress
Of having been diagnosed
With a chronic illness
And trying to care for myself
With the best advice available,

I am a criminal.

My crime is having selected a protocol for myself
Which lies outside of what is USA "approved".

Technically, the compassionate doctors
Who have assisted me
Are also at risk.

I import and inject a vitamin solution,
Approved for my condition,
25 years ago by the meticulous Germans.
It is still routinely used for my condition there.
It is not sanctioned in this country.

Fortunately the courts are clogged.
The jails are full.
My "crime" falls below the radar screen.

But why on earth do we add unnecessary burdens
To the already stressful process of
Just caring for one's own health?

Bring Back Common Sense II

I am angry.

I somehow contained my anger
And got philosophical in that first musing on this topic.

I notice, however,
That when I talk about it with others,
My voice gets louder and more strained,
The tears are not far behind,
And I find myself warning my audience
of one or two or three,
"Don't get me started on this."

Don't get me started on a system
That is insane, that makes me wrong,
That makes compassionate doctors wrong
Not out of any concern for my health.

Something has become more important than my health
And has allowed common sense to be trashed.
Are the pharmaceutical companies afraid
For the success of an alternative approach?

That's the only thing that makes sense to me.

And there is something deadly wrong about that.

Bring Back Common Sense III

Today, Dr. Dean Ornish,
Eminent cardiologist,
Went to Congress.
He testified that his life style change program
Should be as worthy of Medicare coverage
As a heart bypass operation.

For $7000
Change your life with guidance, protocols
And a year of support.

For $50,000
Endure a heart bypass.

A simple economic equation —
Spending on prevention and saving on cure
Makes sense to me.

Sadly, it is apparently not that simple.
The number of entrenched interests
That stand in opposition
Is enough to make me sick!

July 23, 2001

LOOKING FOR THE SPECIAL DOCTOR

When there is no cure,
You doctors have to be special people.
We know how to find you
We have your names and numbers
We talk.

For us, your support is one link to sanity
In our confusing world.
You may be suspect if you prescribe with Western assurance
And pretend that "the only treatment we have"
Is automatically what's best.

You get a high rating for being aware that there are options,
Some of which you didn't learn about in medical school.

What's most appreciated is that you listen, listen, and listen
To our ideas, our fears, to what we know about our condition,
About what works for us, and then...
Offer the best of who you are and what you know.

I seek a partner in exploring my new terrain,
Many partners, in fact.

A Desperate Search Ended

In 1997, when I was diagnosed
Of an incurable, yet manageable, chronic illness,
I took a three-year journey
Into the worlds of the hopeful —
Those whose experiences had given them reason to believe
That there were some answers.

Having no doubt that cures do come from some unlikely places
My curious nature was driven
By my need to be whole.

I tried what the first doctors ordered,
but the prescription seemed incomplete.
So, I got the mercury out of my teeth,
and I'm still getting it out of my system…
I sang hymns in Portuguese and drank herbal hallucinogens
Until two in the morning, dressed in white.
I was stung by bees to strengthen my immune system
I cleaned out my colon from the residue of years
And listened to evangelists for fresh juice and raw foods.
I placed magnets in my shoes.
I wore a pulsing device on my chest
Until I wore it into the swimming pool.
When I wore a second one into the swimming pool,
I figured this treatment was not meant to be.

(continued)

As the stress of the search
Became a burden of its own
I gradually learned to trust a treatment,
And a life,
That was right for me.

I do feel better.
I have a routine of my own.
It's quite enough.

After all,
Being "whole" is really an inside job.

On Leadership

Leadership is not easy
I'm finding that out
As I take a stand for myself
Against the nay-sayers
And for my own healing protocols.

Being a leader in any venue
Makes one a target
For projections and fears
Oft expressed in terms of put downs.

You spent how much getting the mercury
Out from under your crowns?
You aren't taking the approved drugs?

Imagine…
I'm just experimenting leading myself.
Or, perhaps finally trusting mySelf to lead.

ON LEADERSHIP II

Trusting myself — finally!
That's the key to leadership
Of any kind anywhere.

Trusting myself to go into the unknown
With the conviction
That my Self is strong enough
To withstand attacks
To let the naysayers have their truths
While holding to my own
And being open to its evolution.

I'm going to have to practice more
If I am to lead for better health care.

Healing is Not Just About Medicine

"I'm going to get better."

Out flowed these words
As I slipped off the reflexologist's table
Surprising myself with a new and gentle
Certainty of spirit.

I've said them before
Always knowing deep down
That whatever most needed attention in my being
Hadn't yet been addressed.

The phrase "I'm now willing to heal",
Or one of its many variations,
Is the universal test.
Can you say it and feel it at all levels of your body —
Without doubt or hesitation?
If not, you've still got work to do.
So I've known, for so many years.

That day I was touched by grace.
Perhaps the pay-off of a painful journey,
Or, just because my time had come.
There really doesn't have to be a reason.

That day, and since,
I've been touched by grace.
Now, every cell in my body
Says, **"Yes."**

STRESS AT
HOME

YES, IT'S TRUE

I was in denial about
Stress at home.
I'm not anymore.

❋❋❋

Chronic illnesses have a way of
Turning up the volume on lurking problems, and...
Adding others.

❋❋❋

In our king size bed
There's plenty of room
For both of us to sleep alone.

CREATING MORE CHOICES

There is stress in my marriage.

Stress is no good for me.

I find myself seeking a very fine line
Between two extremes:
Sacrificing my health to the relationship, or,
Learning my role in attracting and being
debilitated by
This that I call "stress in my marriage".
It's a daily cost/benefit review.

Here's a new thought…
Since "stress" is basically self-imposed,
I'll put in my order for clarity
About other choices I have

I think I have more than two.

Trying Something New

A friend encouraged me to dialogue with colors:
"Experiment talking with your less-than-conscious self."
She suggested green, blue and purple as an example.

While I love those colors,
I was not too interested in the idea.
Yet, I woke up at 3:00 in the morning
And felt compelled to write.

I wonder if I would have been equally alerted
If she had picked mauve, tangerine or lime.

Dialogue with Colors

Green, blue, and purple remind me of
My bruises on the outside
They come — they fade away.

Red, black, and iridescent orange
Remind me of the colors of
My bruises on the inside.
They have settled in and still hurt.
How shall I encourage <u>them</u> to fade?

On Healing and Growing

When I was a child
I married a child.
There was one complicating wrinkle.
I was 50 and he was 53.

I'm now discovering that my healing is
Critically linked to my growing up.

It's also related to his growing up.

Unattainable Expectations

The man I married
Wanted a kind, gentle, thoughtful, attentive wife,
Like the mother he always wished for
I am the third who failed to deliver.

I, too, wanted a kind, gentle, thoughtful attentive partner
Who would really see me for who I was.
Like I felt my mother never had.

It was painful to recognize
That I had to be that partner for myself first,
And not burden anyone else
With those unattainable expectations.

Beyond the Platitudes

The state of being where
I'm OK as I am, and you're OK as you are
Is a goal worth pursuing.

However, I suggest to myself that
My being OK with me, despite your shitty criticism
Is a wonderful place to start.

And my being OK with you being full of shit,
And not accepting you are full of shit
Is a next step.

Even my being OK with you thinking I'm full of shit
When I refuse to accept that I'm full of shit.
Takes me further.

So when we are both OK with our shit
And content allowing it in the other,
We may finally reach that desired state of being:

OKness with ALL that is,
Because that IS one of the ways it is.

RELATIONSHIPS ARE HARD

If one can listen
With compassion and curiosity
And forego the blaming,
A committed relationship calls out
For each to grow.

"That's nice advice.
What a wise woman you are,"
I briefly applaud myself.

But can I hold this compassion and curiosity
Despite the gnawing pain
And create enough space to ask and answer
My personal call for growth?

ALLOW IT ALL

IN THE SPIRIT OF

10,000 JOYS

and

10,000 SORROWS:

Some days... I feel black, blue, and broken

Some days... I feel sad and depressed

Some days... I feel totally joyous

Some days... I feel enraged and angry

Some days... I feel at peace.

THE SECRET OF LIFE

IS TO ALLOW IT ALL

LEARNING THE LESSONS

Some People Just Don't Get It

I feel compelled to admit
I am one of those who didn't get it.

I read many times that the beneficent forces of the universe
Will knock louder and stronger
Each time you refuse to listen to what you need to hear.

I now know I wasn't really paying attention
To many, many, things.

So, I got the two-by-four to the head
In the form of a chronic condition.

One of my doctors put it very succinctly:
There is only one strategy here —
Change your life or die.

Not too much wiggle room there.
I guess it's time to hit the books and learn the lessons.

TRILOGY
ON THE NEED TO BE PURE

I. ICE CREAM

I had a large bowl of ice cream.
I'll know tomorrow if it was worth it.

It wasn't.

When will I learn that choices
For "long term feel good"
Serve me more than for
Short term need and greed?

II. A Whole Pie Is Not the Solution

The discipline of healing is hard fought
It requires breaking old habits
Of body and mind.
Let me remind myself that "I do choose to be healthy."

Such a Universal Power Mantra
Needs to be backed up by
Real, honest to goodness,
Aligned action.

Up until recently,
When I really felt great
I would go to the health food store,
Buy a fruit pie, and eat the w-h-o-l-e thing.

And then — I would feel bad the next day.
(Something about pleasure and reward
hooked up with celebration and food.)

Today, when I again felt great
Up surged that familiar urge to buy a pie.
This time, I said, "No!"
And with it came a very clear "Yes"
To feeling great EVERY DAY.
Perhaps something is being rewired at the core.

III. Pure Confusion

I don't want to be pure!
I want my ice cream!
And...
I want my pie!

The consequences are becoming more clear —
Eat sugar and feel bad,
Eat vegetables and feel good.

However,
I'm noticing I don't like to do what others tell me I should.
I'm noticing that I don't even like to do what I tell me I should,

Maybe if I listen hard and
Let my body tell me what it needs,
And maybe even let my mind cooperate,
I could align the fundamental facts
With a new fundamental choice.
Sugar just doesn't work for me
And I choose not to have it.

Getting out of the game of
Self-imposed shoulds and rebellions
Is not a piece of cake.

The View Is How Different?

The pickpocket looks at the saint
And sees only her pockets.
Any building I enter
I see only the restroom signs.

Once inside, I notice how narrow are the stalls
And how non-existent are the bars.
It never mattered before.

Through the lens of one's "condition"
The world is viewed differently...
Totally!

What an education in perspective! It makes me wonder what really important information about the world and myself I am not seeing. Only my minor "condition" is one of being recently disabled. My major "conditions" are being white, over 60, married, and a little bit outrageous.

Heavy Metal
(It ain't the music)

I am in detox.
Not for heroin, or crack cocaine
But for the mercury, lead and copper that
Live in my body and interfere with my nerve conduction.

I figure it's a 50 year build up.
I don't have another 50 years to get back to zero.

Dramatic action is called for
Water, Kale, Cilantro and Chard, Selenium and C
Flush them out through my kidneys
Exacerbating my symptoms.

It's called getting worse before you get better,
The darkness before the dawn, "the healing crisis".

It's comforting to know the phenomenon has a name
And that the name refers to something temporary.
Because it isn't any fun.

Too Much of a Good Thing

I'm noticing my tendency to overdo.
When I feel good, I want to do more —
Finish some work, exercise, take on a new project,
Clean out my closet or drawer, go grocery shopping
And then… I'm tired.

I am perhaps using the reserves of yesterday
To push too hard today.

What will it take to learn to STOP
After a little work, a little exercise,
A little project, for a little rest?

The Essential "Off"

My mother has no off button.
She needs to be useful
Until the day she dies.

In fact her definition of 'ready to die' is
"I am no longer useful."
She has already engaged me
As the one she will trust to pull the plug.

I, of the next generation
Am slightly more aware.
I know that I have an off button.
I watch myself standing before it
Inviting myself to make a courageous move
Yet unable to break the family pattern.

What's my definition of 'ready to die?'
I'm not sure.
I am clear that my inability to do
What my mother knows naught about
Brings me closer and faster to
The day it will no longer matter.

I Think There is a Lesson Here

Today I actually pushed my "off " button.
I lay down with two magazines I wanted to peruse.
I wandered through the pages at my own slow pace
And enjoyed the journey.

It was a different quality of time than I experience
When I "take on" the articles listed on my To Do list.
That's work, albeit relaxing, when I finally get to it.

This was pure enjoyment.
Nothing to do.
Nowhere to go.
And when I got up, I briefly walked without a limp.

On the Need to S-L-O-W Down

I conclude that
R U S H I N G
Is one word which no longer
Belongs in my vocabulary.

The activity
No longer serves my good health.

Getting my body to agree
Is not such an easy matter!

MULTI-TASKING MUST GO
(just like rushing)

Today, walking out to my car,
Holding some packages in one hand,
And a glass of water in the other,
I fell. The glass broke, gashing my hand.
Emergency room, here I come!

My doctor said: "AND WHERE WAS YOUR CANE?"

Good question!
While I don't always need it for balance,
I do need it to keep myself from carrying
Too many things at once.

KNOWING OR DOING?

My Knowing comes from a different place
Than much of my Doing.

Now that I am beginning to be able to tell the difference
Perhaps I can interrupt the automatic rush to the Doing,
Settle in with the Knowing and
Make better choices.

LESSONS EVERYWHERE

When I went for a massage
Ruth worked with my right ankle.
She said, "The energy here feels kind of dead."
I replied, "Yes, this is my 'bad leg.'"

She offered me a suggestion,
"'Bad leg' sends a self-fulfilling message to your body.
Why don't you say , 'This is a very good leg,
It just has issues,
And I am learning from those issues.'"

We laughed and I entertained a new idea.

She noted the ankle energy responding to that thought.

WOW! I need to remember in the darkest days that All parts of us respond to love and appreciation.

> **Note to myself:**
> *There is a wider application here.*
> *I have a very good spouse.*
> *Right now, he just has issues.*
> *And, I am learning from those issues.*

I NEED NOT BE ALONE

If I make my husband
The only source of my strength
And he fails me,
I am pretty vulnerable.

I have perhaps placed my tender self in hands
That have much more to do in the world
Than to care exclusively for my needs.
It becomes no one's fault but my own
When I become disappointed, sick or sad as a result.

I NEED NOT BE ALONE II

Let's think this over again.
What are the multiple dependencies I can claim
That will sustain me and nurture my existence?

What a great question — and
What fun exploring the possibilities
In nature, in creative arts, in music and meditation
In special teachers and friends, in spirit,
Always remembering that
The spouse is but one possible source among many.

Meditation Meditation Meditation

Meditation Meditation Meditation

Meditation Meditation Meditation

Meditation Meditation Meditation

Meditation Meditation Meditation

Meditation Meditation Meditation

Meditation Meditation Meditation

Meditation Meditation Meditation

Meditation Meditation Meditation

It's not been easy to sit and "do nothing"
Just listening for that still, small, voice
Which is me, and
My salvation.

PATIENCE

They tell me it took my whole life
To get what I have.

So, although I believe in
The possibility
Of Spontaneous Healing,
It will probably take the rest of my life
To master nourishing myself
And letting go of old ways.

LOSSES

A QUESTION

Loss and limitation

Come to all of us

Sooner or later.

Is this now for me

My sooner?

Or my later?

GOOD MODELS

I joined my 87 year old mother
And my 92 year old aunt
For lunch one day.

My mother laughed about her hearing aid
Determined not to be like those other old folks
Who blame their lack of hearing
On everyone else's lack of volume.

My aunt noted the new presence in her life
Of what she called "the borrowers."
They are the spirits who
Take things temporarily
And then, in their own time,
Return them to a different place.

Both are good models for me.
My aunt still walks the mountain,
But drives half way and walks the flat.
My mother is cutting back on her tennis,
"Two games a week instead of three, and
perhaps ping pong sooner than later."

One element of successful aging it seems
Is to adjust to one's limitations with grace.
At 61, with a chronic illness,
I'm starting on the same journey
A little earlier than they.
May I be equally graceful and patient with myself.

PAINES CREEK TRILOGY

I

Today, I had high hopes.
I went to Paines Creek beach.

My plan was to sit for a while,
Then cool off in the water,
Alternating that routine
To keep my body cool.

Within 5 minutes I felt the heat
I once loved and relished,
Attack my nerves and disable me.

Low tide was too far away to
Comfortably walk and
Cool myself down.

Fearful of not getting home,
I left…

Very sad

Another loss

I want to cry

I did.

PAINES CREEK TRILOGY

II

After the tears,
I crafted another accommodation
To the reality of this particular illness

Tomorrow,
I'll go to the beach
At high tide
In the early morning
When it's still cool.

PAINES CREEK TRILOGY

III

I wouldn't be here this early
But for an accommodation to my condition.
Cane in hand, I limped down to the shore,
Insistent on swimming in my ocean.

But notice!
How quickly joy replaces sadness.
Being in the ocean alone
At a wonderful, peaceful, tranquil time of day,
Is thrilling!

A couple watching me said,
"How much we enjoy you
Taking such pleasure exercising and
Nurturing yourself in the water."

I received two gifts:
Loving appreciation from perfect strangers,
A new time to enjoy my beach.

Another Note to Myself

ALL RIGHT, ALL READY
I'LL TAKE MY CANE!

With feet that are numbing
My walk is slower and a little less stable.
Since I can still manage,
I've proudly resisted my cane.

However, others need a signal
And I ought to provide it.

Drivers are more patient with me at the crosswalk
When they see my cane
Crowds part and create a path for me
When they see my cane
People stare less at my drunken gait
When they see my cane.

All of this being true
I actually feel safer in the world
When I have my cane.
So ALL RIGHT, ALL READY!

On Deservedness

I first got my handicapped pass
When I was walking easily for short distances.
I looked quite able bodied…
At least for the 20 yards it took to walk from
The handicapped spot into the building.

Being a responsible citizen, I feared "they"
Would think me cheating the system.

The guilt was short lived.
I now limp like a pro the very first step.

How is it that I must visibly limp to feel deserving?
Am I more dependent on what others think
than what I know to be true?

Therapy Swim

It's been years since I've played tennis,
I can no longer run,
Although last night I dreamt myself jogging comfortably.

Since I no longer walk any distance
I go to "therapy swim" and exercise
With the "retired, over 70" crowd.

While all of them are older than I,
Some are fatter and some are thinner.
Most walk faster and
A few walk slower.
Some attend for the swimming
And others for the talking.
They seem to be a network of support for each other
And, amazingly, even for me.

Norm introduced me to my Tai-Chi program
Harry and Dolly invited me to Barbershop
June suggested where I could read my musings
And find a writing group.
All greet me by name, even though Norm forgets,
And comes out with Sara or Barbara.

These "old" people are not old in spirit
They are living full lives
With spunk, irreverence, and joy.
What great models for me
As I try to do the same.

No Regrets

"I'm ready to retire." and "No regrets"
I'm surprised at how I feel this morning.
With these two ideas co-existing comfortably.

I thought I might come to a place
Where I would know that it was time
To give up the work I love, and still
Be full of regrets,
Kicking and screaming,
Sad and angry at
The hand of cards life had dealt me.

Instead, it feels comfortable and right to move on.

My daughters are giving me a priceless gift.
They are learning to be good stewards of
What I most care about.

And they are doing it out of love for the work.
How much better can it get?

TODAY

Maybe just for the moment

I feel the need to cry

I think I will.

THEN THERE WAS SEPTEMBER 11

For hours, even days, it is a bad dream
That didn't really, couldn't really,
Not in my wildest dreams really,
Have happened. Each morning I wake up,
Feeling normal for a moment — until I remember,
It's not a dream and it never was.

I cry, and I cry, and I cry
For the reverberations of pain
Set off in our world — by four air bombs.
For the many, many, many losses to families
Across the nation.

This grief uncorked, flowed in my direction, too.
Over the last few years, my health,
My marriage and mySelf
Had taken their own hits.
These assaults, not fully attended,
Were hungry for the tears due them
And grateful for the end of silence.

I wonder why it took a national tragedy
Of such immense proportion
To allow me to mourn my own losses.

GAINING PERSPECTIVE

ON KNOWING

I attribute the incredible stress of the year after my diagnosis
To the compulsive searching for answers from others.

Some residue of childhood baggage
Had me thinking of myself
As a person who didn't know…
Which made me at various times the perfect counterpart
To a mother who was very certain about all things,
To a spouse who likes to think he knows more than most,
To doctors who are trained by Western medicine
To know better — always.

Now that I am more trusting of the clarity of my own knowing,
I am a less than congenial dancing partner
As daughter, patient and spouse.

And I feel relieved — most of the time —,
My own answers are working for me.

SELF AWARENESS

There are no techniques to learn
No answers to seek, but one —
Self awareness.

Who am I?
What do I desire?
What is my experience of myself engaging with life?

If I can be true to myself
I know where I am with others.

LISTENING TO ONESELF
IN UNLIKELY PLACES

Deep in the MRI machine
I was left alone with my thoughts.
My mind, as it so often does,
Started mentalizing.
My body began to tense.

Fortunately I'm learning to ask
"What poem is trying to emerge?"
Then I relaxed.
My body wisdom kicked in,
Three brilliant musings flowed forth with abandon.

Now to remember them
Once I am out of this cave.

THE AFFIRMATION TRILOGY

I

When I leave my own small world,
I get a new and refreshing perspective.

My husband and I had moved back to the town of my younger
years.
An old boyfriend and his wife were about to retire and move
south.
I decided to say "hello" and "goodbye"
After not being in touch over a space of 12 years.

He was a special man in my life at one time.
And I a special woman in his.
We had a great visit.
His e-mail the next day confirmed this.

"You are soooo beautiful.
Your grey hair becomes you,.
I hope you will come and visit us down south."

It was the "soooo beautiful" that got me.
That affirmation meant a lot.

Although I have learned over the years
To affirm for myself
What I know to be true
I wonder that my husband can never find those words
I would so love to hear from him.

THE AFFIRMATION TRILOGY

II

Interestingly enough,
I'm now hearing and enjoying
New and delightful affirmations.

From my mother,
My brother and sister-in-law,
My new friends who love my poetry,
My old friends who care about me
My daughters,
My nephew,
My new healer team
And always, my clients.

It's nice to live in a wider world
Able to let in
All that is there for me.

THE AFFIRMATION TRILOGY

III

A needy child of any age
Seeks affirmation compulsively
And it is never enough.

I assert that everyone needs
Encouraging confirmation
Of their existence.

As a 62 year old recent "grown up"
What has become newly clear is a distinction
Between the seeking to fill unfillable needs
With specific words and gestures I demand from others,
And the relishing of available affirmation from others
That I have been first able to give myself.

YES

Friends who love me

Take care of me

And, I allow it.

Reframing Anyone?

My friend and I were saying that
On SOME days, life SUCKS.
Preferring to have a different view of events,
She asked: "How can I hold that idea
As not so depleting and draining?"
We imagined a fish sucking…

At least it gave us a giggle.

DIFFERENTIATION, FINALLY?

It's OK with me

That it's not OK with you

That I think how I think,

Love what I love,

Am who I am.

YESSSS!

TRILOGY
ON LISTENING

I

As a person who needs to know and understand,
Listening to whatever wants to show up unannounced
Can be disconcerting.

A fearful self, a critical self, or a linear self
Provide no welcome mat for a visiting muse
No matter how essential the message.

II

What may not at first make sense,
May be a truth in a language yet undecipherable.

III

One day in the woods,
I gave myself permission to listen.
A scream erupted — actually more than one.
Beautiful, natural, pure, and deep.
"Who I am" was there.
I heard.
And I understood.

MY OWN VOICE

The burdens and stresses are falling away.

As each slides off my shoulders.
It turns into a poem.

The process started naturally one day,
As if the universe were guiding me
To a new, and more healing way, to respond.

I call it happiness.

Releasing the worries
And finding the wisdom
Of my own voice.

May 1, 2001

A Hard Truth

Afflictions ultimately heal.

Skipping the despair doesn't work.

Power of Perspective

I'm beginning to see that

The healing power of Truth

Is found somewhere between

The tears and the laughter.

TODAY

Watching the Process

DAY ONE

Today
I found two parts of me sparring.
"I don't want to live," was challenging
"I do want to live."
No one was winning.

DAY TWO

I called a friend.
She let me cry.
"No more fighting," she said,
"Relax into living."

DAY THREE

In human beings
Doubts arise.
Allowing them is essential,
Choosing anew is available,
Friends are indispensable.

ACCEPTANCE

I have what I have.
It just is.
You wanna make something of it?

Sure…
I'll make it OK for now.

Everyone Needs Support

In my MS support group
People listen respectfully
To experiences they themselves share and
Few others understand.

I now know why in wider society,
Such groups of "likes" exist
And why they sometimes appear to be
Exclusionary, and even discriminatory.
It takes one to know one.

I wish this act of listening deeply,
Seeking to understand,
Were more routinely practiced.

POETRY READING

I took the next step
Went down to the Bookstore
For the Open Mike poetry reading
And read some of these musings.

I got an appreciative response
Encouragement to publish.
A stranger gifted me his book
Of self published poems

Three high school students,
Read their generationally wise perspectives
On a world breaking down.
I admired their courage.

As a new writer, I found these young people intriguing.
I inquired about their process.

"These just come to me, and I write them down," one said.
"It's good to have a vehicle to express my thoughts," the other
added.

I couldn't agree more.
Sharing poetry across generations is a very cool thing.

TRILOGY
On Regrets

I Tuesday

I feel at peace.
To have no regrets
Is a very comfortable place to be.

II Wednesday

Actually, I do have one regret.
That while living with a diagnosis
And very few visible symptoms,
I was not sufficiently motivated
To make the changes in my life
For which this condition calls.

Not taking something seriously
Until it is too serious to ignore
Is a choice that looks very different in hindsight.

III Thursday

Hmmmm. Interesting that
Being both with regrets and no regrets
Are somehow still perfectly compatible
With feeling at peace.

Writer's Workshop

One Sunday, I went to an afternoon workshop
The premise: Written expression can be a tool for healing.
Deep in the beautiful Berkshires
Six middle-aged women talked, wrote, and shared.

When I got tired, I lay on the couch and took a nap.
The teacher asked us to write one final reflection
On our afternoon together... Here's mine.

There are many nurturing places.
One, I discovered in the Berkshires
Lying on a couch with strangers
Who could be friends
Able to let my own soul speak.

I want to remember to give myself time and space
For this kind of nourishment —
Always available if I seek it
And — if I allow it.

WATCHING THE PROCESS II

In a dream last week
I went to a mountain top
And received a powerful blessing.

Night after night since,
I have dreamt of myself running,
The way I used to,
Joyously, freely, easily.

What does this mean?
Are there deeper forces aligning
To ground my deeper healing?

I'll keep watching.
This is getting interesting.

October 8, 2001

In the Silence

In the silence
If I wait long enough
I feel myself SAD

In the silence
If I wait long enough
I feel myself ANGRY

In the silence
I no longer have to wait so long
To feel myself
BE MYSELF
Whatever way I am,

And to ultimately rescind my vow of silence.

Making Sense

I no longer fight my chronic condition.
I receive it as a gift–with gratitude.
These words just flowed out,
Totally surprising me!

This unplanned adventure has succeeded in
Calling forth my own hidden Heroine
To face a mysterious challenge.

Seeking and creating paths
To unknown destinations,
Discerning which guides to trust,
Accommodating detours, wrong turns, loneliness and fear,
Accepting downs and ups, humor and grief along the way.

Until one day
I emerge —
Walking forward —
With Clarity and Hope as new companions
The five-year journey is starting to make sense.

I wonder what the next five years will hold?

ACKNOWLEDGEMENTS

This first edition, originally published in 2002, never started out as a book. So I have to thank old friends in Washington DC (Jill and Evelyn), and new friends in the Pioneer Valley (my business group and my health care team) who validated my expressions as having meaning to others beyond myself. They encouraged me to publish my musings about my own process just as they occurred to me.

Alan, Amy and Deborah gave me the confidence that our business was in good hands and I could attend to my healing process wherever it took me. My 87 year old mother has become a model of support and encouragement for me as we grow to older adults together. My healers/supporters to whom I have dedicated this volume have deeply affirmed my discoveries and opened the channels for the activation of my own healer/knower.

My friend and longtime editor, Jill Davis, was the one who first read my efforts. When she said, upon reading the first 18 musings, that the editor's pencil in her mind never once appeared, this was validation beyond belief. I looked at my work with new eyes and kept going. My husband Alan offered to format the manuscript for publication with his special artistry and attention.

I must thank my husband in a deeper way. He was a protagonist in this journey—as I have been in his. In 1997, he was also diagnosed with a serious illness—prostate cancer—from which he has successfully recovered. In my judgment, we have both been "defended" in such a way that we needed to be the pit bulls for each other to crack open whatever has held our patterns in place. (That is another set of musings.)

I am grateful above all, that he has always been willing to grow with me, and I with him, and that we have worked hard to live up to what is so easily violated these days—" marital commitment." If we should ever deactivate that commitment, I believe we will do it together for the right reasons. I am proud of both of us for that.

Martha Johnson Gilburg
January, 2002

About the Author

At the time of the publication of the original printing of this volume, the author was living with her husband at the base of a mountain in the Pioneer Valley of Western Massachusetts. She was soon to fully retire from her business as founder and co-owner of Growth Dynamics, Inc. a coaching and consulting practice, principally based in Washington, DC. Committed to the process of healing and regaining health during these years, she put priority on nourishing activities of writing, painting, and swimming. This was her first book.

Please visit
TIME for YOU: www.taketimeforyou.net
Phone: 413-532-2579
Email: martha@taketimeforyou.net

Other Books by Martha Johnson

Why Not Do What You Love! An Invitation to Calling and Contribution in a World Hungry for Your Gifts (2010)

Musing Along the Way: Pain, Persistence and Purifying Waters, Volume Two: The Years 2002–2008 (2011)

CPSIA information can be obtained at www.ICGtesting.com
Printed in the USA
LVOW041536291011

252654LV00002B/5/P